Love Yourself

Kill Depression

BY

N. C. ENESHA

Other Books by N. C. Enesha:

1. **The Last Pagan**

http://www.amazon.com/gp/aw/d/1515293629/

2. **Senior Dating Guide**

http://www.amazon.com/gp/product/B00S3O4AWO/

3. Creative Imagination Guide

https://www.amazon.com/dp/1523831731/

Email: ncenesha@gmail.com

This book is informational and educational on how to use love for yourself and love for others to kill depression

ISBN-13: 978-1539631750

ISBN-10: 1539631753

DEDICATION

This Book is dedicated to Chukwu, and Dr. Ugochukwu, Dean and Head of Cross River State University of Technology's School of Basic Medical Sciences, Okuku Campus, and his family

INTRODUCTION

Love is the universal law of happiness and success. Without love, gloom and depression set in. Love is the infinite space on which creativity thrives. Although the word "love" has been overly desecrated, it is the law that governs creation. It is love for creativity that made the Creator create the universe and all that it contains. You were created with love, so to lack love for yourself and love for others is to be like a fish out of water; hopeless, gloomy, hateful, depressed and wishing to "end it all" for yourself, even though love is an easy and beneficial emotion to express for your own good and the good of others.

What does it take for you to love yourself?

Nothing but self appreciation.

What does it take for you to love another person?

Nothing, other than the appreciation of the infinite truth that you are a person because of another person.

Love begets love and all the good things of life. Love makes you godly; it is the eternal and immortal link between you and your

Creator. To love is to positively play God. Without love life is bleak and difficult. Every good deed is derived from love, which power radiates joy and happiness in both the lover and the loved. Love rules your destiny, it is inevitable that you love and be loved.

Love is the heart and soul of the Creator, so if love increases in you, you are in harmony with your Creator, and this will enable you to happily continue to create for humanity, in accordance with the rule of love, the foundation of all creations.

Love has the power to clean you of depression and diseases. The power of love is limitless, even the workings of the universe is based on the love of the Creator.

Disease, ill health, bad governance and corruption, disasters, petty quarrels, wars and selfishness are all implicated in lack of love. Imbue yourself with love and love for others, and be free from depression. Verbally or in your mind say the below mantra as many times as you can everyday and your life will change for the better:

"Every minute of every day, I love myself. Every opportunity I get, I share my love with others. And I am getting better and better in many ways every day."

Holding onto thoughts of negative experiences is a sign of weakness. Memories of sad experiences do not die natural deaths, you have to kill them with the realization that you still have more and better chances than you have lost. Survival demands that you muster enough strength to let go sad thoughts to create space in your mind for happiness and joy.

Love never flourishes in a mind full of negative thoughts; rather love dies because there is neither happiness nor joy in your mind to feed it. Love dies of emotional wounds on you or on another person. Yet love can resurrect a dead love.

However, when love dies, it is important that you do not succumb to sadness, rather look inward and love yourself enough to keep fit, both in mind and body by believing that you are born to love and be loved, and that better times lie ahead.

Love attracts happiness and joy to feed on, and love can also hurt seriously if you do not realize that it can hurt. Wherever there is joy, sorrow lurks around, waiting for the opportunity to pounce on your heart, but you have the capacity to withstand all the challenges that may come your way. Just know that as you can look back on your tears and laugh, you can also look back at your laughter and cry.

I also want you to note that life is a lonely journey if you have no one to love, and no one to extend a hand for you to hold. Enliven your journey by creating love within you to share to fill the emptiness you feel. Remember that the pain that maintains a broken heart can lead to mood swings and other depressive symptoms, and that type of depression is self-inflicted. Suffering for a loss or imagined inability is not penance, even though penance amounts to suffering on purpose unlike the self-inflicted suffering associated with depression.

The hardest part of creating and sharing one's love is the ability to forgive both yourself and your offender. No heart is made to break, yet hearts break for lack of love.

Friend, you cannot love yourself and still experience low self-esteem and depressive symptoms that precede and indicate the approach of depression. This morbid condition can result from a feeling of loss, self-doubt and guilt, plus the erroneous belief that people consider you worthless. Why? Simply because you do not believe in and love yourself any more.

Self-doubt usually stems from lack of love for self, fear, or failed attempts at achieving a goal. But if you love yourself, and that goal is important to you, should you give up? No, rather you should try again and again to win the goal for yourself, become successful and garner love from people—success attracts love. Giving up on ideas and endeavors brings about low self-esteem, which in turn leads to fear, self-hate and depression.

Friend, you ought to love and believe in yourself, and believe also in something too; your mind requires an anchor lest it drifts away. And since your mind feeds on appreciation, a "thank you" received is lovely and builds confidence in you, so acquire as many "thank yous" as you share your love with others each day of your life.

You are actually a person because of another person, so love yourself and love other people too.

And when you make yourself useful to a neighbor and receive a "thank you;" with a heart full of gladness and joy, also thank your Creator who used you to help another person: Say, "thank you Father, for making it possible for me to share love." Every good deed is a share of love, just as your creation was a share of love by the Creator.

Thankfulness

A feeling of thankfulness and appreciation increases love in both you and your helper. And because your Creator is your infinite benefactor, whenever you receive a "thank you" for your lovely deeds, be happy and thank your Creator for making it possible for you to be helpful. Your life will be better if you are always thankful for the blessings of life. Anyone who does not show appreciation for a good turn defiles an expression of love.

If a "thank you" does not brighten your heart in appreciation of the privilege you received to be of help to another, it means your deed was not born of love, but of some reason, even though love is never in agreement with reason. This is an in-harmony against the state of true love, which is universal and unpolluted by any form of bias.

A mind that is in harmony with the Creator gives thanks for life, for water, for light and ultimately for love of self and love for others, and this mind is always thankful for the love of the Creator and those of other people towards it.

Love has a place in you; it is a universal law that governs and directs your destiny. If you destroy or jettison love from your being, you will ultimately deny yourself the true desires of your heart. You are created to be a co-creator with the Creator of the universe, but you cannot fulfill your destiny without love. Depression is the absence of love, use love for yourself and love for others to cleans yourself and rule your destiny.

Read on to help you learn how to kill depression with love for yourself and love for others. Love is the conqueror of all life's undesirable situations, including depression and distorted thinking!

Love Yourself: Kill depression

What is distorted thinking?

It is a mindset that convinces you that what might not be true is true just because your mind says so. Below are 15 distorted thinking mindsets that you should know about to help you love yourself and others and live a depression free life:

1. Filtering: You take the negative details and magnify them while filtering out all positive aspects of a situation.

2. Polarized Thinking: Things are black or

white, good or bad. You have to be perfect or you're a failure. There is no middle ground.

3. Overgeneralization: You come to a general conclusion based on a single incident or piece of evidence. If something bad happens once, you expect it to happen over and over again.

4. Mind Reading: Without their saying so, you know what people are feeling and why they act the way they do. In particular, you are able to divine how people are feeling

toward you.

5. Catastrophizing: You expect disaster. you notice or hear about a problem and start "what if's". What if tragedy strikes? What if it happens to you?

6. Personalization: Thinking that everything people do or say is some kind of reaction to you. You also compare yourself to others, trying to determine who's smarter, better looking, etc.

7. Control Fallacies: If you feel externally

controlled, you see yourself as helpless, a victim of fate. The fallacy of internal control has you responsible for the pain and happiness of everyone around you.

8. Fallacy of Fairness: You feel resentful because you think you know what's fair but other people won't agree with you.

9. Blaming: You hold other people responsible for your pain, or take the other tack and blame yourself for every problem or reversal.

10. Should: You have a list of ironclad rules about how you and other people should act. People who break the rules anger you and you feel guilty if you violate the rules.

11. Emotional Reasoning: You believe that what you feel must be true-automatically. If you feel stupid and boring, then you must be stupid and boring.

12. Fallacy of Change: You expect that other people will change to suit you if you just pressure or cajole them enough. You need to change people because your hope for

happiness seems to depend entirely on them.

13. Global Labeling: You generalize one or two qualities into a negative global judgment.

14. Being Right: You are continually on trial to prove that your opinions and actions are correct. Being wrong is unthinkable and you will go to any length to demonstrate your rightness.

15. Heaven's Reward Fallacy: You expect all

your sacrifice and self-denial to pay off, as if there were someone keeping score. You feel better when the reward doesn't come. Culled from http://livelearnevolve.com/15-types-of-distorted-thinking/

References:

Beck, A. T. (1976). Cognitive therapies and emotional disorders. New York: New American Library. Burns, D. D. (1980). Feeling good: The new mood therapy. New York: New American Library.

From mood swings to depression

Tony and Gloria dated happily until Gloria began to suffer mood swings as a result of pantothenic acid (vitamin B5) deficiency. Her confidence and self esteem began to dwindle as she continuously picked at every of her supposed flaws, creating a devastating cycle that developed into self pity, low self esteem and irritability.

Irritability is a common depressive symptom in which simple disagreements frequently turn into heated arguments. A depressed person is more likely to be aggressive in an argument, because they defensively feel that they are right. Even little things like difference of opinion can set off a fight. A depressed person's level of patience and tolerance depletes quickly leaving them feeling tense, nervous, excited, irritable and ready to fight anyone and everyone, which is why they find solace in solitude.

Tony was surprised. Unfortunately, he could not handle Gloria's new attitude. He did not know that Gloria was suffering from depressive symptoms, and that what was required of him was understanding and the display of more love for her.

Gloria wondered where she went wrong. How was it that Tony, with whom she shared her life, became somebody she argued with most of the time? Why did things change from how they used to be to open hatred of her by Tony? She had no answers.

The truth was that it didn't have to be that way if Gloria's psychology remained unaltered by biological changes the couple could not handle. To make matters worse, sufferer and partner were not aware of what was the matter. Disagreements and arguments became the other of the relationship until a break up. Heartache, especially for the one whose mood swings and several other depressive symptoms engendered the break up, followed.

Tony did not know that a simple lovely Text message could have began to heal Gloria, whom he loved very much before her moods threw spanner into the wheel of their love affair. He did not know that love can cure depression.

For instance, an appreciation Text message filled with love could have had Gloria feeling loved and confident about herself again, but Tony was rather angry and distanced himself from his sick lover. Believe me, love filled Text messages work positively on the mind of a depressed person; it is better than talking in person, especially if the depressed is angry with you.

If Gloria had received love filled Text messages from Tony, she would have started to feel better and confident in herself, and her self esteem would have rebounded, and she would have started to love herself as she felt loved. Love can remedy any awful condition, including depression.

What is Depression?

Depression is a mental state characterized by a pessimistic sense of inadequacy, a despondent lack of activity and lack of love for yourself. It makes a sufferer feel worthless and inferior to all and everything he or she could have done. A depressed person, as the name suggests, is held down by this morbid condition from a level of activity to inactivity. He is prone to negative thoughts about himself and everything around him. His thoughts begin to guide his actions, which in most cases are inaction, making the person moody and hateful. If not treated, depression can lead to thoughts of suicide, and its commission.

Let me say it in-your-face that it is your responsibility to save yourself from living in a lost state of mind, without direction, unfulfilled and bitter, because only you can put yourself down by accepting negative thoughts or negative outside influences. To pull yourself out of depression, you must love yourself and believe that you can achieve any goal you work hard at, consistently smiling at all challenges. The first step at fighting and wining depression is to get up, get out and begin doing something useful for you or for other people.

Believe that challenges thrive on bitter and negative thoughts. Above all, note that our lives depend on the love of one another and that if you do not love yourself it is impossible to love anyone or accept their love.

Depressed persons always find faults in themselves and in others, which ultimately makes them withdraw into their shell, with their minds filled with the negatives of the past, regurgitating the faults or inabilities of their parents and everyone else as excuses for labeling themselves worthless.

However, the good news is that it takes just doing the opposites of the foregoing to begin to love yourself so that you can begin to forgive and complement others wholeheartedly. A sincere "good morning" with a genuine smile to someone is a show of love, which you can only give if you also love yourself.

Is Depression Curable?

Yes, depression is quite curable if you recognize that you have it and make effort to love yourself and make up your mind to fight it by accepting that you are loveable and therefore ready to make changes necessary to ward off depression, not by way of self-medication with anti-depressants, which can really adversely affect the functions of your brain. Rather, it is safer for you to see a doctor or a qualified health practitioner to determine whether or not you are actually depressed, and whether your particular type of depression requires medication or psychological therapy.

If it is your loved one who is experiencing symptoms of depression, ensure that they do not self-medicate with anti-depressants, rather lovingly encourage them to see a doctor.

The below article by Gregory Pack throws light on the use of anti-depressants:

7 Facts about Antidepressants the Pharmaceutical Companies Don't want You to Know

Are SSRI's Beneficial or Detrimental?

1) SSRIs cannot cure depression - Nor are they designed to. Selective Serotonin Re-uptake Inhibitors are designed to block the body's natural re-uptake of serotonin so that more serotonin is available to act on

receptors in the brain thereby producing a mood lift. Unfortunately the low serotonin levels associated with depression are not the cause of the condition but rather the result of excessive stress being placed on the mind. SSRIs can provide some welcome relief for sufferers but are by design only beneficial to temporarily control extreme symptoms, not cure depression.

2) SSRIs users commonly experience relapse rates of up to 80%. SSRI exhibit such alarmingly high relapse rates because they focus on altering the "chemical imbalance" in the brain while ignoring the

cause of those imbalances; therefore when the medication is denied, serotonin levels again fall and the depression relapses. In only approx 20% of cases the mood lift effects of depression medications are sufficient to push them past a minor stressful event.

3) SSRIs are highly addictive often resulting in dependency. Since the FDA approved Paxil (Paroxetine) in 1992, approximately 5,000 U.S. citizens have sued its manufacturer GlaxoSmithKline. Most of these people feel they were not sufficiently warned in advance of the drug's side effects

and addictive properties. It's not the ingredients in SSRIs that are addictive but rather the feelings they invoke by increasing serotonin. Sufferers become "addicted to the happy feelings" caused by the medication, a scenario that often leads to long term use and increased probability of serious side effects.

4) SSRIs side effects include aggression, violence and suicidality. A 2004 FDA docket states "Strong obsessive suicidal thoughts emerged after Prozac treatment. The serotonin system enables us to dismiss normally fleeting and transient suicidal

thoughts and prevents us from acting on aggressive impulses. Excessive augmentation [increasing serotonin] may render us unable to dismiss these thoughts, leading to uncharacteristic obsessions." In data from Sertraline (Zoloft) paediatric trials submitted by Pfizer, "aggression was the joint commonest cause for discontinuation from the two sertraline placebo-controlled trials in depressed children."

5) SSRI Discontinuation Syndrome: A condition that occurs during or following the interruption, reduction or discontinuation of regular SSRIs. The most

common symptom being "Brain Zaps" which are said to defy description for whoever has not experienced them, but are described as a sudden jolt likened to an electric shock originating in the brain itself, with associated disorientation. These symptoms are considered to be caused by the brains attempts to readjust after such a major neurochemical change in a short period of time.   In January 2007, Hugh James Solicitors in the UK commenced litigation against GlaxoSmithKline on behalf of several hundred people who allege withdrawal reactions through their use of Seroxat (Paroxetine). The issue at the heart of this action claims Seroxat is a defective drug in that it has a natural tendency to cause a withdrawal reaction.

6) SSRIs prescribed to children can be a lethal combination. Currently the only SSRI that is FDA approved for depression treatment in children and adolescents is Prozac; all others have been banned from paediatric use as their safety and efficacy have not been proven. Despite this in 2002 there was 10.8 million antidepressant prescriptions dispensed to children under the age of 17 by U.S. physicians with less than 1 million of those being for Prozac.   In March 2004 the FDA proposed that the

makers of all antidepressant medications update the existing black box warning on their products' to include warnings about increased risks of suicidal thinking and behavior, known as suicidality, in young adults.

7) The Fastest, Easiest and Most Effective permanent depression treatment is NOT medication. Excessive stress results in depression, yet the quantity and intensity of stress one experiences is not determined by any particular external circumstances but rather by ones perception of how those circumstances will impact their life. In

addition the body's natural reaction to stress is to activate serotonin re-uptake; hence when you reduce your stress the serotonin levels return to normal, boosting your mood without medication.

By utilizing specifically designed subconscious techniques it becomes quite simple to create a mindset based on positive perceptions in only a few days, thereby breaking the cycle of stress, anxiety and depression - permanently. - - - - - - - - -

and the author biography remains unchanged. Gregory Park is the Director of Research at Depression Perception.com, a company whose commitment and dedication to the research and development of advanced depression treatment techniques is proving exceptionally beneficial to many people. Their techniques work by re-writing the mind's negative thought patterns with positive new perceptions, thus removing the cause of depression. Submitted by Gregory Park on Tuesday August 21, 2007.

http://www.articlealley.com/article_204 945_17.html

How does human depression compare with economic depression?

Depression in economics refers to a long-term economic state characterized by unemployment and low production, low levels of trade and investment, inflation of prices and rise in crime, just as clinical depression is characterized by inactivity, lost man-hours and low or lost income, lack of purchasing power, inability of the sufferer to communicate properly, and irritability. If you are feeling moody and irritable, go for a checkup so that if you are depressed, treatment could begin in earnest to nip this morbid condition in the bud. The earlier a depressed person begins to receive treatment, the better the chance of remedying the condition.

How does a depressed person feel?

When you begin to experience feelings of gloom, inadequacy and, at least, three of the below symptoms:

1.   Insomnia, chronic sleeplessness, or hypersomnia, inability to stay awake

2.   Substantial changes in weight—weight

loss or weight gain

3. Domineering feelings of guilt, loss, worthlessness and helplessness

4. Day long chronic fatigue

5. Lack of concentration or inability to focus on anything

6. Fidgetiness, anxiousness or feeling under pressure

7. Feeling dull all day

8. Inability to experience pleasure, anhedonia.

9. Haunting thoughts of self-destruction and death; better show love to yourself and go see your doctor because, aside from vitamin B5 (pantothenic acid) deficiency, those are the symptoms of depression.

Even though a normal person can naturally feel depressed for a loss, love for yourself and self preservation will normally jolt them out of it to set goals and joyfully work towards its attainment, while a depressed person will normally set no goals, rather he or she will bicker and bitch and look for faults and excuses with which to deepen his or her sadness, which in turn culminates in the feeling of worthlessness.

Depression is like total darkness that induces melancholy and apprehension. A depressed person is always afraid of the future. He or she usually creates in their mind an atmosphere of gloom and wallow in it. He or she is both the prisoner and self-jailer. A jail break is only possible for a depressed person if they accept the reality of their condition and fight back with love for yourself and the right professional care.

However, even though temporary depression due to certain happenstances is human, you must not let yourself drop into a state of anhedonia, so severe as to require clinical intervention. Love for yourself is the antidote, just shower love on yourself; set a goal to break free and become successful, wholeheartedly work at it with positive creative imagination and persistent determination, and your mind will be better occupied by the expectation of success. Do not jail yourself in the dark room of hate and depression.

Let me tell you this: The biggest mistake someone who has depressive symptoms makes is idle away his or her time on the bed to avoid social interactions.

While it is true that what causes depression is different for different people, the symptoms are similar even though how individuals respond to them are different too, making it extremely difficult to generalize treatment.

However, the first line of treatment is to accept that you have depressive symptoms and develop a strong willpower to cooperate with a qualified Ayurvedic doctor for your treatment.

It is a proven fact that orthodox medicine provides palliative relief, meaning that you must continue taking the drugs for controlling the disorder throughout your life time. On the other hand, Ayurvedic herbal treatment in combination with psychological therapy gives better result and cure by my personal experience; though psychotherapy alone has proved more effective with depressive symptoms arising from personal problems such as separations and social or work anxiety.

How do you recognize signs of depression?

It is natural to become depressed following a loss. But at what point of feeling depressed for a loss can it be said that clinical depression has set in? For instance, if a relationship crashes, it is normal to feel sad, lose sleep, appetite and even feel guilty. But is any loss too costly to warrant self-hate to a degree of thinking about suicide?

If you feel angry and unhappy for a loss for more than one month, it is a sign of depression. But you can reverse your mood by saying several times a day: "I love myself, this loss is not as important as the least thing I can do with my lovely life." This statement of fact and the feeling it will stir in you is a bulwark against melancholy and depression. Always place yourself above any situation or happenstance.

Note that failure to promote love for yourself will lead to loss of interest in normal daily activities, especially disregard of activities you once enjoyed. You can begin to feel guilty, hopeless and worthless followed by over sleeping, only to wake up and indulge in crying spells. Soon also you will begin to notice the deterioration of your memory, and unexplainable weight loss or gain, coupled with tiredness and speaking in an unusual low monotonous tone.

From the foregoing, the signs of depression can be confused with everyday feelings that many people experience due to a loss or failure to achieve a set goal, so do not overlook such feelings if they become ongoing. Always reassure yourself: "I love myself, this loss is not as important as the least thing I can do with my lovely life."

Self imposed absence of feelings

Exhibition of lack of feelings is just an excuse with which a depressed person hopes to escape from negative emotions and fears. Most depressed people numb themselves hoping to escape from the pain they feel. And what this does is isolate the sufferer and make worse the condition.

So please do not mask your trouble with self imposed absence of feelings, for yourself and for others. What you should do is love yourself enough to inform your loved ones about what you are going through, so as to enlist their support and love, because love begets love. If you fail, your depressive symptoms will increase until they completely take you over and lock you up in a void no one can reach.

I say all these things to implicate you if you or your loved one is experiencing any of the mentioned symptoms. But how can you be sure that what you feel is depression? *Is what I feel not just ordinary blues?* Please, I want you to know that your best chance of knowing whether what you feel is depressive symptom or not is to go see your doctor. And if you are diagnosed to be depressed or heading towards it, the very first thing you must do is to love yourself enough and decide to fight depression with everything possible at your disposal

Below are common types of depression:

Medical experts have identified more than ten different types of depressions, some of which I list and explain below:

Major depressive disorder

This is a serious mental disorder that takes a person over completely, which is why it is called (MDD) Major Depressive Disorder. Sufferers wallow in a sense of despair and weakness. This type of depression is evident when symptoms remain continuous for two weeks without abatement.

Mild Chronic depression also known as Dysthymic depression:

Dysthymia is evident when you continuously suffer moodiness for two or more years. This type of depression, in spite of its long duration, is not usually as severe as Major depression, which completely disables the normal routine of life of a person.

Mild chronic depression

This is usually hereditary, and the symptoms are generally ignited by stress.

This mental disorder is not reserved for adults alone, it can happen to children. Medical experts are unanimous in stating that about two percent of global population will suffer mild chronic depression in their life time.

Bipolar disorder

Manic depression or bipolar disorder is a complex mental condition characterized by moods of extreme sadness and extreme happiness. Bipolar 1 and Bipolar 2 are the two kinds of this type of depression, which can be very severe in nature; it does not go into remission like some other depression episodes. It must be treated to get a cure. If not treated early it can metamorphose into psychosis and the patient will become delusional, suffer paranoia and hallucinations, a condition in which patient may become unable to take care of themselves. Medical experts have identified bipolar depression to commonly occur in people of age fifteen to twenty-four years. The cause of this mental disorder is yet to be identified.

Atypical depression

This is a momentary mental state

characterized by gloomy episodes. It is usually common with people who had experienced depression earlier in life. Unlike other types of depression, an atypical depression sufferer can

intermittently experience sudden feelings of happiness as reactions to good turn of events. With the right type of treatment this type of depression can be remedied quicker than most other depressions.

Psychotic depression

This is a state of depression so severe that the person loses contact with reality and suffers a variety of functional impairments, because he is no more able to distinguish between hallucination and reality. He can suffer both auditory and visual hallucination and consider them realities. For this condition, treatment is usually long term and continuous.

Melancholic Depression

This type of depression is usually triggered by an event or a loss, it is considered a mental disorder. Even though it can also be considered a symptom of major depression, it can be hereditary too. If you have this problem, you can remedy it by showing love to yourself by quickly seeking treatment from your doctor or a health care professional.

Postpartum depression

Unlike other forms of depression, postpartum depression is easy to cure. It usually occurs to some women immediately or several weeks following child birth. The symptoms are sadness and hopelessness, due mostly to hormonal changes and the physical trauma of the delivery of a child. Research shows that postpartum depression affects one in 1000 women worldwide. This morbid condition needs treatment; without early treatment it can lead to psychosis.

For some moms, this health disorder occurs immediately after giving birth while for others it can take up to one or more months after delivery for the following symptoms to begin to occur: However, please note that the symptoms outlined below only become issues of concern when they become regular:

1. Feeling not free and caged.

2. Feeling neglected

3. Self condemnation for whatever goes

wrong

4. Constantly annoyed and irritable

5. Easily tearful

6. Feeling of loneliness even when with family and friends

7. Feeling of anhedonia, in ability to feel pleasure.

8. Neglecting of the new born baby and desiring to commit suicide.

All the above feelings sap energy from the sufferer of postpartum depression, making it difficult for her to lead the normal joy filled life of a nursing mother. She will find it difficult to concentrate or remember things. Even her sleep will be impaired, and each time she manages to grab a short sleep it will be marred by fearful dreams. All that being said, postpartum depression symptoms are not in the above order for every woman, but suffering from three or more of any of the above symptoms is enough reason to hurry to your doctor without delay; and that will be love for yourself.

Depression in Teenagers

Because of emotional, hormonal and physical changes teenagers go through, they are less resistant to depression, which can be considered normal growing up mood swings, but such state of mind becomes a problem to take care of if a teenager is habitually moody, inactive and irritable. Although teenage years can be very difficult period of human development when inevitable changes, both emotional and physical, take place in a human being, it is important to differentiate such teenage crisis from depression. The following are depressive symptoms you can mistake for teenage crisis:

* Extreme distortion of sleeping and eating habits, especially too much sleep.
* Self condemnation and hopelessness
* Sudden withdrawal from social activities

and friends

* Malcontented attitude and inclination to suicide

One reason why teenagers become depressed is due to peer pressure, e.g., a teenager can become depressed because of how he or she is perceived and treated by mates at school. It is worst for such a teen if there is no love at home to go back to. Make your teenager feel loved by you, so that they can confide in you for reassurances, to keep depression at bay.

Is Depression only caused by feelings of loss or an unfavorable event?

No, depression can be caused by multiple other factors. Medical experts say that clinical depression is the outcome of a process that began a long time before its manifestation, usually derived from genetics/biology or psychology. One factor or a combination of factors can contribute to the sickness.

Whether your child or a loved one is going through teenage crisis or is actually depressed, the first step towards improving the condition is the show of love. Love has the power to make your child cooperate with both you and the doctor or a health care professional who provides treatment for his or her condition. And if you are personally suffering from any of the above types of depression, shower love on yourself, set a time frame to get well, because you have a grand plan to achieve a goal for yourself in the service of humanity.

Diet and Depression: Foods to avoid

People all over the world get depressed from time to time in their life time due to some unfavorable happenstances, lack of contentment, or vitamin B5 deficiency. For instance, research in the United States indicates that about half of the population bear the risk of suffering depression of some sort before the end of their lives.

Does this mean that not all depressions are emotional? The answer is yes. Research has also indicated that some foods can cause some people to feel depressed in spite of the so called blood/brain barrier. It states that what you ingest can actually derange your thinking to a certain degree. In some cases, extremely.

Below are foods you must avoid if you are feeling gloomy or you are diagnosed as depressed

* Foods rich in dairy hormones can create gloomy moods or worsen depression. For instance, foods such as cheese and other dairy products are not good for you if you have mood swings or you are depressed, because poultry animals are usually impregnated with hormones for quick growth. Most of those hormones instigate wild mood swings

* Caffeine intake can lead to anxiety and depression. It is an established medical fact that regular use of caffeine leads to inability to sleep; or even chronic sleeplessness, and lack of sleep leads to daylong low energy, fatigue, irritability and aggressiveness.

* Alcohol abuse can cause depressive symptoms. What alcohol does when you ingest it is depress your nervous system, and if depression or mental disorder runs in your family your chance of developing depression or even psychosis becomes heavy.

* Sodium and fluoride. If you consume too much salt you will receive enough sodium to deteriorate your neurological system as well as your immune system, thereby making you liable to negative emotions. Also, fluoride, according to several studies, has the capacity to cause cancer. It is said to be able to damage your pineal gland, which in turn lowers your IQ.

* Refined sugar is not good for you, because it can trigger depression symptoms. This happens because, even though your brain uses lots of glucose, refined sugar spikes your insulin levels leading to low blood

sugar and this naturally affects your brain adversely. Your starving brain becomes anxious; your mood begins to swing towards depression.

* Glutens are gelatinous proteins found in grains, but wheat is the chief carrier of these proteins. The issue with glutens is they are difficult to digest, so they build up in your blood stream, and because they are excitotoxins like glutamate, aspartate, and cysteine, three amino acids that excite our neurons and cause mood swings.

Unfortunately, people who experience symptoms of depression and those who are already depressed consume these foods. If you suffer mood swings, or you are already depressed, it's a step in the right direction to avoid these foods.

Good foods for alleviating depressive symptoms.

It is love for yourself if your diet contains nutritious ingredients, so that your general health condition, especially the health of your brain is well maintained. I am talking about consuming wholesome organic foods prepared at home as against ingesting fast or processed foods. Several researchers have found that lack of the right nutrients in your diet can predispose your brain to an imbalance that can lead to depression.

The foods you eat can affect your body either negatively or positively, especially the functions of your brain. Certain foods are known to help improve brain functions; below are foods you should make part of your diet to either bar or eliminate depressive symptoms:

Beans

Folic acids enable neurotransmitters to function effectively carrying messages between your brain and your body system, and beans are very good sources of folic acids.

Vitamins and Minerals rich foods

These include spinach, tomatoes, green veggies, broccoli and whole wheat products.

.

Fish

Fish and its oil are used to cure and reduce depression, because they contain omega 3 fatty acids that build your neurotransmitters and improve serotonin secretion to regulate your moods positively. Doctors put depression patients on omega 3 fatty acids.

Antioxidants

Antioxidants help your body, especially your brain to eliminate free radicals that can cause the oxidation of your brain tissues. Antioxidants are found in oranges, potatoes, carrots, dark chocolate, spinach, peppers and lignan seeds that inhibit HSD enzyme which may reduce the stress hormone Cortisol.

Manage light to relieve Depression

Descartes, a famous philosopher of yore,

called the human pineal gland the "principal seat of the soul." The Occultists call it the "third eye." However, modern science has proof that these claims are not far from the truth considering the position of the pineal gland in your brain and its activities. The pineal gland seats in the middle of your brain at the same level as your eyes. Although this organ is very small, rice-sized, it plays important roles in the regulation of your sleep/wake cycle, mood and feelings.

Did you know that your thought process, pattern and how they make you feel is governed by the pineal gland with its production of melatonin and serotonin, the hormones that regulate the quality and duration of your sleep, plus your physical performance and stress levels,

In order to positively regulate your sleep, energy levels and mood, there are two proven ways to activate your pineal gland for utmost production of melatonin and serotonin, neurotransmitters involved in sleep, depression and memory:

a. **Sun Gazing:** Get up and go outside and take a couple of seconds gaze at the

Sun to activate your pineal gland to produce adequate serotonin. Do this before the Sun becomes harsh to look at.

b. Sleep in a dark room: You can relieve depression by keeping away from artificial lights after Sundown to avoid confusing your pineal gland into thinking that it was still day-time and thus continue to produce serotonin, which in turn distorts your sleep/wake cycle. Sleep in a completely dark room, without backlit from phones, tablets and computers, to promote the production of enough melatonin by your pineal gland.

Exercise relieves Depression

Since depression has the capacity to make you sedentary, exercise is one essential means of liberation for a depressed person, who is going through a most draining experience in life, because depression affects not only your emotions but also your physical health.

Depression saps you of energy and ultimately drives you into a state of social isolation in your bed, making it difficult for you to get up and move, even though the weakness you feel is not in your muscles and limbs.

While it is very important to consult your doctor the moment you begin to, for any reason or unnecessarily, feel discontentment mixed with gloom or melancholy, remember that exercise is one way you can personally deal with depression on a daily basis. It is common information that exercise promotes wellbeing by preventing serious diseases such as diabetes, high blood pressure, obesity etc....several researchers report that depression can be relieved with daily exercise.

Did you know that just 30 minutes of exercise done three or five days every week is sufficient to relieve depression symptoms, and that even 10 or 15 minutes at regular intervals is good for short term improvements of your mood?

It's opined by researchers that exercise activates neurotransmitters in your brain to positively affect your mood. Exercise activates endorphins, a neurochemical occurring naturally in the brain and having analgesic properties—it is known as a "feel good" chemical that helps to release tension in your muscles. This chemical also helps you to sleep comfortably by mitigating the actions of the stress hormone known as Cortisol.

Is it therefore true that exercise can cause chemical changes in your brain and body to relieve depression symptoms such as self-doubt, stress, anger, anxiety, hopelessness and sadness? Yes, daily 30 minutes exercise can relieve your depressive symptoms. However, exercise may not bring you a complete cure, which is why it is necessary to show love for yourself and consult your doctor or a qualified health care professional to help you manage your depression. Though I do not propose exercise as substitute for proper medical care or treatment for depression, I advise you to love yourself and begin to make it difficult for depression by refusing to be held down on your bed or sofa; get up and do something for yourself, choose the type of exercise you enjoy most and engage in it every day. When you think about it, it may seem too difficult to get out of bed and exercise, but the truth is you can do it, just love yourself and get out of bed.

It may be swimming, jogging, cycling, brisk walking that you like, just know that exercise of any kind is recommended by medical experts for the promotion of cardiovascular, muscle and your general well being. For instance, the American Heart Association and the American College of Sports Medicine endorsed a regulation for all healthy adults of ages eighteen to sixty-five to engage in, at least, thirty minutes moderate exercise for five days of every week.

However, if you have a chronic condition, or a physical fitness limitation, seek medical advice from your doctor or a qualified health professional before engaging in any sort of exercise. Exercises can improve both mental and physical health. For instance, engaging in aerobic exercises can improve your cardiovascular endurance, the flexibility of your muscle and its strength.

One of the great benefits of exercise is it pumps more blood through your veins, thus, it increases the size of your arteries and this helps to prevent blood clots, or thrombosis. Exercise accustoms your heart to endurance and so it does not find it difficult to pump enough blood, meaning you are not prone to heart attack. If you exercise regularly you enjoy the added benefit of increased good cholesterol and a lowered level of bad cholesterol. Your blood pressure is also lowered as your blood ways are opened up for easy blood circulation.

The best Exercises for Depression

It is not true that any particular exercise is more effective for depression, what I know is that you should pick the exercise you find enjoyable, so that you can do enough of it for the desired effect: to make your brain produce enough endorphins.

Exercises you can do:

Brisk Walking

Swimming

Bicycle ridding

Jogging

Table tennis

Long Tennis or

Dancing

The above exercises are by no means all you can do. Just go for the exercise that you enjoy. If you like, you can join a Club and play different kinds of balls and running sports too. But because depression introverts and isolates sufferers, you should love yourself enough to enlist the assistance of a relative to do the registration in your desired Club for you. You will do yourself a lot of love-favors by being in company of people instead of solitude. If you feel not up to going alone to the Club, get one of your loved ones to escort you.

Exercises wash away gloom

When I first came across this fact, it was a big surprise for me. How can exercise help to regulate my mood; I was feeling very low at the time - I had just lost my first job. Jackson my friend advised me to choose the exercise that I like to make better my depressive mood. And I was surprised that during and after my chosen exercise I felt better. So I looked up "exercise and mood" on Google and found that several researchers have confirmed what I felt. When I exercised, my body released endorphins, hormones that act like morphine to dull sensation of pain and bring about some sort of euphoria.

I asked some athletes how they felt after a competition; "euphoric!" was the answer from almost all my respondents. One of them said, "I feel a "cool high" that is not intoxicating." I asked a medical expert why athletes feel a "cool high" after each practice or competition. He said to me, "they feel high because physical exertions make their brains release endorphins, which act as both analgesics and sedatives creating a feeling of euphoria. It's marvelous that the brain releases endorphins to reduce pain during and following the exertion associated with physical activity that is involved in races and other sporting activities. So it pays to exercise when your mind is heavily burdened, it will keep you busy and make your brain release the 'feel good hormones.' Regular exercise will keep depressive moods at bay."

If you are already depressed, you can use exercises to love yourself and begin to recover quicker than one who is not exercising. Medical experts say that depressed people who combine medication with exercise recover quicker from depression than those who rely on only medication.

Mental and Emotional Exercise

Aside from medication and physical exercise, mental exercise is very important to regain control of your emotions. To help you achieve this, repeat the mantra below verbally or in your mind several times a day:

"Every minute of every day, I love myself. Every opportunity I get, I share my love with others. And I am getting better and better in many ways every day." Memorize and act the above quotation. Practice what you say and you will easily begin to love yourself and others for your own good, because depressive symptoms cannot comfortably cohabit with such positive thoughts in your mind.

Believe that as long as you love yourself and others, you will definitely, with positive thoughts and constant effort, deaden negative and depressive thoughts in your mind.

Other Books by N. C. Enesha:

1. The Last Pagan

http://www.amazon.com/dp/1515293629/

2. Senior Dating Guide

http://www.amazon.com/gp/product/B00S3O4AWO/

3. Creative Imagination Guide

https://www.amazon.com/dp/1523831731/

Email: ncenesha@gmail.com

ABOUT THE AUTHOUR

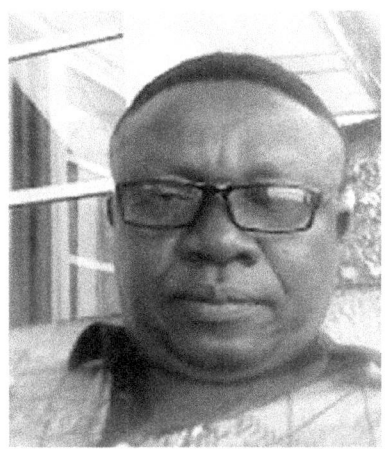

N. C. Enesha (1955 - date) lives at Port Harcourt . He is an Expert Author with Ezinearticles.com. . When he is not busy writing, you will find him under a mango tree in his house, ordaining characters with destinies for his readers to enjoy.

Love Yourself: Kill depression

Love Yourself: Kill depression